Wall Yoga

Supported Yoga Poses for Seniors, Beginners or Athletes for Balance, Strength and Good Posture

Melinda Wright

Reviews for This Book

"By utilizing the support of a wall, even beginners like myself can achieve greater balance, strength, and good posture. The step-by-step instructions are clear and concise, making it easy to follow along and enjoy the benefits.

One of the aspects I truly appreciate about this book is its inclusivity. Whether you're a senior looking to improve mobility, a beginner seeking a gentle introduction to yoga, or an athlete aiming to enhance performance, Wall Yoga caters to all levels and needs. The detailed visual demonstrations further aid in understanding the correct alignment and form."

Patricia R. Morgan, USA

"This book is perfect for beginners and people with some mobility issues and more advanced age. There's no excuse not to do yoga with a book like this one."

Robert M, USA

"I have been scouring for books that can help me reconnect with yoga after a long-standing illness and this is it! Supported yoga with chair and wall poses and photos to help me along. Really glad I gave this a go."

Jessica Birks, UK

"This is a transformative and accessible guide that brings a fresh perspective to the world of yoga. With clear instructions and innovative wall-based techniques, it caters to all levels of practitioners, offering a comprehensive journey to inner peace, strength, and well-being. I loved the fact there are QR codes that take you directly to the very clear videos on how to do these poses as well as a great recipe for no-bake carrot cake! This book is a must-have for anyone seeking to enhance their yoga practice!"

Nathalie, UK

I am impressed with the quality of this book. Everything is easy to follow and the videos are very helpful to make sure I do the technique correctly.

Marianne, UK.

Contents

Foreword

I strongly recommend this book "Wall Yoga" for anyone who is starting Yoga or perhaps is a senior with less confidence in the practice. As with her other books, she gives very pragmatic advice on which are the best exercises to do, in this case, with a wall. There are clear and concise instructions with clear photos for each exercise. The videos via a QR code are also very helpful.

Melinda is a wonderful Yoga and Pilates instructor who uses her wealth of experience to explain the most effective methods of approaching yoga practice. I have been very fortunate to have been able to attend her classes regularly for years and know firsthand how successful her methods are. Her warm and engaging style really motivates you whether in person or via the book.

As a GP, I am increasingly seeing patients with symptoms associated with lack of exercise or poor nutrition. I feel we would all benefit from following Melinda's advice and exercises.

Thank you, Melinda, for writing such an excellent helpful book, guiding us to improve our well-being! Also many thanks to Sytske for being such an inspiring model despite her current circumstances, and to Joan the skilled photographer.

Caroline Oliver

MBBS FRCGP

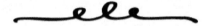

Chapter 1
Why Choose Wall Yoga

Would you like to become more flexible and have a good range of movement with joints that move freely? Would you like to improve your balance, agility, and mobility in order to prevent falls and become stronger? Would you like to feel relaxed and happy during and after your workout? Then Wall Yoga is for YOU!

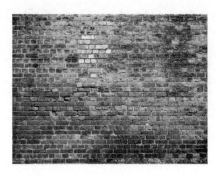

In order to be agile and thus move freely we need to have 3 things: **strength, flexibility,** and a degree of **fitness** in order to be able to move. You are in the right place for developing these here in this book. You know that you need to move however, it may be challenging to get started.

Wall workouts are particularly beneficial for beginners and seniors as they can be performed in a standing position. Getting up or down from the floor is not required for wall workouts. The wall also provides additional support and stability. The incidence of falling or losing your balance is significantly reduced and therefore it's safe for many people.

If you are already fit or are an athlete looking for a challenge the wall provides this too. Using the wall enables us to challenge ourselves more in many poses. There are also many inversions we can do such as headstands and handstands against the wall which invigorate us and strengthen the upper body.

You may start with just a few of these wall poses and build up your strength and confidence. You can enjoy the many benefits of Yoga while staying safe and free from injuries.

You will benefit from my decades of experience as a Yoga and Pilates instructor, group exercise teacher, and personal trainer. I have been helping people to keep their bodies strong and flexible for over 30 years.

Direct links with the added ease of QR codes take you to videos of most of these exercises.

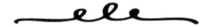

Chapter 2

Prepare to Start

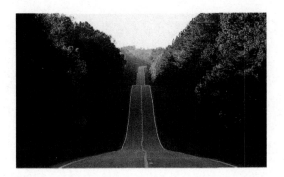

Clothing

Wear comfortable clothing that makes it easy for you to move in. Not too baggy and not too tight. You are welcome to be barefoot, however, if you prefer to wear shoes make sure that they allow you to move freely and are not too bulky. If you wear socks, make sure they have a grip on the bottoms so that you do not slip.

Wall or Surface

You will need something to lean on. It can be a wall, a pole, a door, or a large wardrobe.

Make sure that if you are using a pole it is sturdy enough to lean your whole body weight into.

If you are using a door be careful that you secure it or lock it so someone doesn't come through it from the other side causing you injury. In some of the exercises, a railing or bar would be suf- ficient to provide support.

Use a non-slip mat on the floor in front of your wall surface.

For a recommendation of my favorite mat see my website: https://melindawright72.wixsite.com/website

Hydration

Make sure you are well hydrated by drinking a glass of water or juice. Keep a water bottle handy so that if you become thirsty during your workout you can easily reach it. Do not work out on a full stomach. If you do need to eat something right before exercising fruit is the best choice as it is very easy to digest and provides you with instant energy.

Connect with your Body

This is best done via your breathing. As soon as you bring your awareness to your breathing, a natural link between your mind and body is established. If you cannot breathe during an exercise you are working too hard. Ease off a little and take a deep breath before continuing.

Notice how your body is feeling and stand up tall with good posture. Check in with your body regularly throughout your workout being sure not to overexert yourself or work through pain. If you feel pain, stop. Undue stress on the body can lead to fatigue so exercise within your limits and build yourself up slowly.

Be Patient

It takes time to get the results you are hoping for. They definitely do not arrive overnight. Yoga and Pilates are highly effective ways to improve your overall well-being and fitness however require a commitment to doing the exercises consistently. Even 10 or 20 minutes is enough at first and you will soon be able to enjoy the benefits that come from a regular practice.

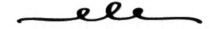

Chapter 3

Simple Wall Poses

Wall Stand

- Stand with your heels against a wall.

- Let the whole back part of your body be in contact with the wall ie, your calves, glutes, shoulders, and even your head if possible.

- Lastly, lift up your arms with your palms facing each other. Keep your shoulder blades on the wall.

- Take at least 5 breaths here.

You may find it quite challenging to stay glued to the wall.

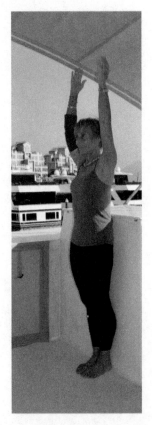

This pose is good for your posture and it also reveals your shoulder flexibility. In the photo shown, the wall doesn't extend high enough up the body. You also may find it difficult to find a wall in your home that is free. If so, use a door or a wardrobe to lean up against.

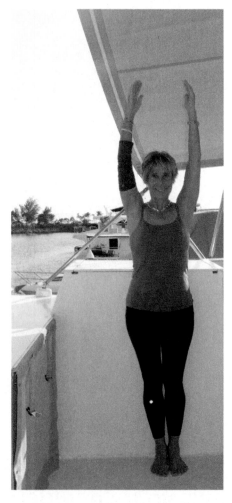

One of the best ways to keep an eye out for any changes in your posture is to stand up against a wall. Over time our posture can become more forward-stooping if we are unaware of it.

Try to keep your whole body sticking to the wall. Do you have to tilt your head back to get it to touch the wall? If so, this indicates that your chest muscles are tight, which pulls your shoulders forward, creating a bad posture.

Your neck and head are then carried forward too. Try to squeeze your shoulder blades into the wall without arching your back. Pull the shoulders back and down the wall. Keep your ribcage from flaring out by pulling your front ribs towards your back ribs. This keeps your lower back safe and in its natural curve.

You may also practice this exercise lying down on the floor. Perhaps your arms do not touch the floor, indicating tight shoulders. Gravity will assist you in getting your arms over your head without straining your neck.

See a video of the Wall Stand by scanning the QR code below or at the following link: https://youtu.be/rZYc1PKIsa8

Wall Chair Pose

- Stand with your feet about a foot's

distance from the wall.

- Bend your knees and allow your sitting bones to rest on the wall.

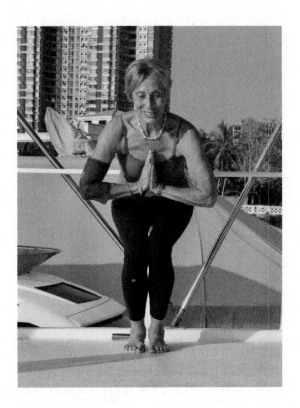

- Bring your back away from the wall so that your body is making a lighting bolt shape with just the buttocks resting on the wall.

- Press your weight into your heels. Hold this chair pose for 5 breaths.

As you can see in this photo, we are using a pole instead of a wall. You may use any firm surface to lean your buttocks on for this pose.

This Wall Chair Pose develops your strength and stamina in the physical realm and your patience in the mental realm.

Make sure you can see your feet. If your knees are covering your toes then you will feel this more in the quads than in the glutes. It is essential to use your glutes in the chair pose as this will strengthen them.

It is common to round your back in this pose. Make sure it is straight!

See a video of the Wall Chair Pose by scanning the QR code below or at the following link: https://youtu.be/U0EDJjz MHMw

Wall Chair Twist

- From the Wall Chair Pose keep your spine very straight and twist your chest to the right side.

- If you can, place your left elbow on your right knee and use it to lever you around in this twist. If your elbow doesn't reach your knee just twist as best as you can.

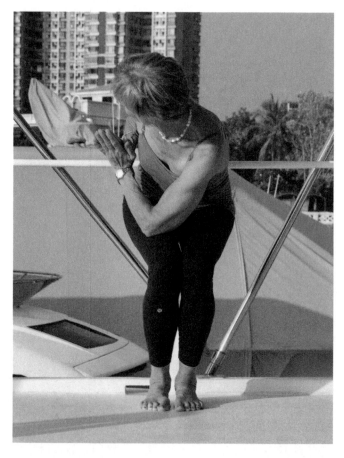

- Keep pressing your knees together and keep both sitting bones on the wall.

- Keep your spine as long and straight as you can while you twist around it like an axis.

- Keep your head in line with your toes. Take 3 breaths here before changing sides.

The wall helps to keep us aligned in our chair twist. Often when we do this pose away from the wall the knees come apart and the spine starts to round. This twist goes deep into the body. It has a squeezing effect on the internal organs and it also trims the waistline.

See a video of the Wall Chair Twist by scanning the QR code below or at the following link: https://youtu.be/49Mms ov1yr4

Wall Forward Bend

- Stand up against the wall with your feet about a foot away from the wall, and hip-width apart.

- Lean your buttocks into the wall as you fold your upper body forward, holding your elbows. Place your hands onto your legs if there

is strain at the back of your legs

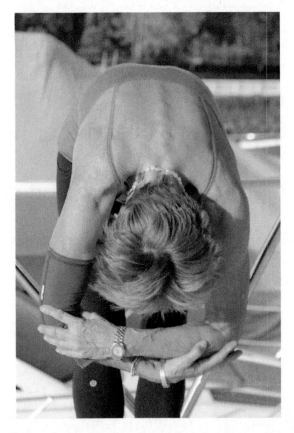

- Bend your knees if this feels better for you or you can choose to
  keep them straight.

- Stay in this pose for 5 breaths or
  more.

- Roll up slowly, vertebrae by vertebrae, until you are leaning against the wall with your whole back.

- Rest against the wall until the blood drains out of your head.

Forward bends are cooling and calming.

They also stretch the hamstrings and lower back.

They also help to release the neck.

See a video of the Wall Forward Bend by scanning the QR code below or at the following link: https://youtu.be/cbt2-71QhHE

Wall Triangle Pose

- Stand with your feet wide open and your hips and back against the wall.

- Turn out your right foot to the right side so that it is parallel to the wall and about a foot away from the wall.

- Turn your left foot slightly inwards (towards the right) and keep your left heel up against the wall.

- Bend at your right hip and reach over your right leg, extending your waist evenly on both sides of your body.

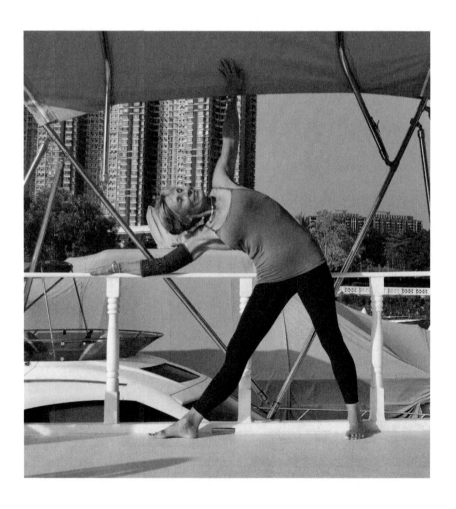

- Take your right arm either down onto your right leg or hold onto something as shown in the photo.

- Extend your left arm up towards the sky.

- Lean the back of your body against the wall, and even your head if you are able to.

- Take 3 to 5 deep breaths here.

In the photo above we are using a railing and some poles instead of a wall. Get creative with your own surroundings and see what will work for you. Try to keep both of your hips and your shoulders on the wall.

The triangle pose is a wonderfully expansive pose for the hips and heart area. With the added benefit of a wall, you will really feel supported. You can lie back against the wall which keeps your hips in a good position and prevents your upper body from leaning forward.

Many people perform triangle pose incorrectly by taking their arm/hand too far down on the leg and this causes the bottom to push back and the spine to curve. Using the wall will help to keep you in the correct alignment.

See a video of the Wall Triangle by scanning the QR code below or at the following link: https://youtu.be/UCzboMqtE0k

Wall Tree Pose

- Stand with your back up against the wall, or just in front of the wall.

- Lift your right leg and place the sole of your right foot against your inner left thigh.

- Press your right foot into your left leg and simultaneously press your left leg into your right foot.

- Lift your arms up over your head and stretch towards the sky.

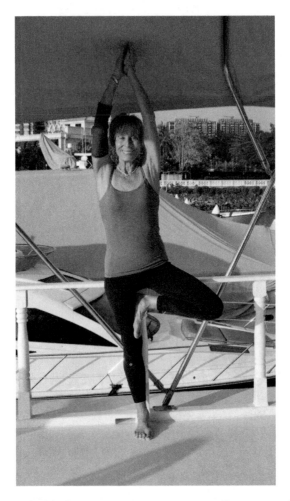

- Hold this tree pose for at least 5 breaths or more before changing sides.

Draw an imaginary line down through the center of your body and try to stay on this line. You may choose to place your right foot closer to the ankle. Make sure that your right foot is not pushing into the side of the left knee, so either above or below the knee is good.

Keep your gaze steady on one spot. Choose something close by that is not moving at first and then challenge yourself to look further away – aiming to eventually look at the horizon. Imagine that you are a tree with roots growing out of your foot deep into the center of the earth. Visualize your root system being strong and stable.

Healthy trees are supple and move gently in the wind. If you hold your body too rigidly here you will feel like your energy is stuck and you may feel tense. The wall will help you to balance in this pose. If you would like to challenge yourself, stand a little in front of the wall and try the tree free-standing. The wall is there as a safeguard to prevent you from falling. Balance poses like this develop strength in your legs, ankles, and feet. They also calm a busy mind. Many of your smaller proprioceptive muscles get to work here, improving your balance overall.

See a video of the Wall Tree Pose by scanning the QR code below or at the following link: https://youtu.be/Ryq3HLbZ-94

Wall Warrior 2

- Stand in front of a wall with the back of your body either touching the wall or very close to it.

- Take your legs wide apart with your toes pointing forward.

- Turn your right foot out to the right side and bend your right knee to 90 degrees. Keep your right foot about a foot from the wall.

- Turn your left toes slightly inwards about 5 centimeters and keep your left leg straight. Keep your left heel touching the wall.

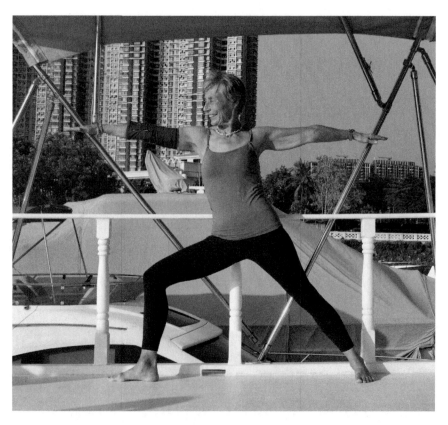

- Lean against the wall if you need

support here.

- Lift your arms out to the sides at shoulder height and gaze over your right arm.

- Take 5 breaths here before chang-ing sides.

You will need to have enough space be-tween your legs so that when you bend your right knee it is directly above your ankle. Bend your knee deeply and point the knee in between your big toe and your second toe, to be precise.

You will be engaging your inner thigh muscles for this. Keep your hips level with each other so that if you were carry-ing water in your pelvic bowl, the water level would be parallel to the floor.

Keep your torso directly above your hips. It is tempting to lean towards the right side. Stay present instead of reaching into the future. Keep your arms strongly extending out to the sides.

The heart and chest are open in this pose as well as the hips. This is a balancing pose and excellent for developing equanimity and staying mindful of the present moment.

It's a wonderful pose to practice outdoors where the grounding quality of the pose will be enhanced.

In the Wall Warrior 2 Pose above we are using poles for support. You can use anything you have for support in your surroundings as long as they are safe to lean on.

See a video of the Wall Warrior 2 by scanning the QR code below or at the following link: https://youtu.be/JxFK7yEEqfA

<u>Wall Hip Stretch</u>

- Stand about a foot's distance away from the wall.

- Allow your bottom to rest on the wall and your back to come forward similar to Wall Chair Pose.

- Bend your right leg and place your right ankle above your left knee.

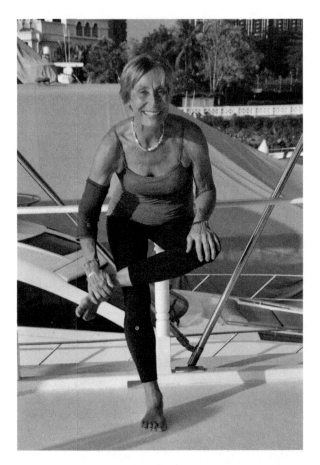

- Push your right knee more out to the side to feel the stretch in your hip.

- Keep your back straight and stay in this stretch for 5 breaths before changing sides.

This pose is a great glute stretch. It is a convenient way to stretch your glutes without having to sit down or get down onto the floor.

The wall provides a firm surface to lean into and helps with your balance in this pose. We are once again using a pole to balance against.

Tight glute muscles can have an impact on your lower back and also may contribute to hip pain.

Keep your glutes and hips flexible by doing this stretch every day!

See a video of the Wall Hip Stretch by scanning the QR code below or at the following link: https://youtu.be/Qnzl6b P3tmY

Download a FREE PDF of a Quick Reference Guide to the Simple Wall Poses by scanning the QR code below or at the link: https://dl.bookfunnel.com/7g5 0s73hdx

Chapter 4

Challenging Wall Poses

Wall Half-Moon Pose

- Stand with your legs about 4 feet apart with the back of your body and your heels against the wall.

- Turn your right foot out to the right side keeping it parallel to the wall and about a foot away from it.

- Lean over to the right side, bend your right knee, then put all your weight onto your right foot.

- Lift your left leg up, keeping it parallel to the floor.

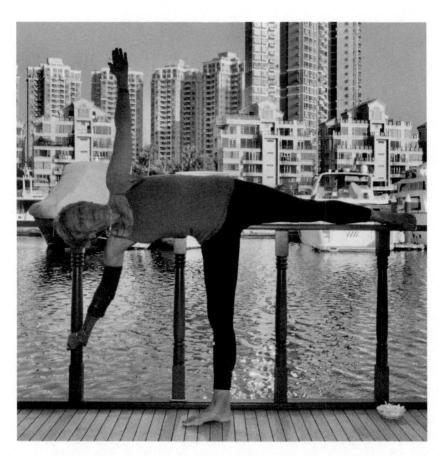

- Flex your left foot and point the toes forward. Keep your left heel on the wall.

- You can use a brick for added height under your right hand or hold onto a support as shown above.

- Stay in the pose for up to 7 breaths.

This pose can be very enjoyable especially against the wall as you get help with your balance.

You can just lie back on the wall. In the photo, we are using a railing which is a good height for this pose.

Get creative and use what you have around you to support yourself in these poses.

See a video of the Wall-Half Moon Pose by scanning the QR code below or at the following link: https://youtu.be/LAUE1P Qgj-M

<u>Wall Side Angle Pose</u>

- Stand against a wall with your legs wide apart.

- Turn your right foot out to the right side keeping it about a foot from the wall. Place your left heel against the wall.

- Bend your right leg at 90 degrees

and lean towards the right leg. Place your right elbow on your right leg.

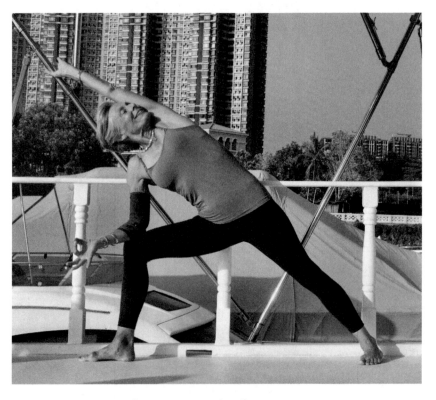

- Stretch your left arm over your head next to your ear. Make a diagonal line with the left side of your body.

- Keep resting your buttocks and your back against the wall and stretch the left side of your body from your left heel to your left fingertips.

- Hold this for 5 breaths or more before changing sides.

You may choose to grip onto a pole or a railing if you have one near you. This pose is a strong stretch for your left side and it is strengthening for your legs. Having the additional support of the wall helps you to really lengthen and relax into this pose without having to worry about your balance.

See a video of the Wall Side Angle Pose by scanning the QR code below or at the

following link: https://youtu.be/LqCjtGV
6KDM?si=a9Ai3DF6Vg1croEz

Wall Sun Warrior

- Stand up against the wall with your legs wide apart and your feet facing forward.

- Turn your right foot out to the right side and keep your left heel on the wall. Bend your right knee at 90 degrees.

- Take your arms out to the sides, then extend your right arm upwards. Take your left hand onto your left leg.

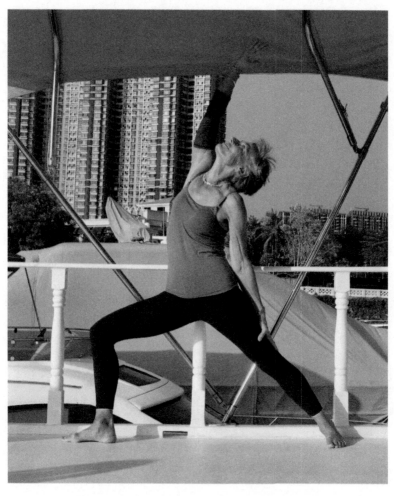

- Curve over to the left side. Reach

as far down your left leg as you can.

- Feel the stretch on your right side as you bend over to the left.

- Hold this pose for 5 breaths or more before changing sides.

We turn our faces up towards the sun in this beautiful sun warrior pose. Feel grateful for all the warmth and life that the sun brings.

See a video of the Wall Sun Warrior by scanning the QR code below or at the following link: https://youtu.be/g1uFTS1-cXY?si=NdX3GNvHXlALJ-8Y

Wall Dancer Pose

- Stand next to a wall or railing for support, with your right side facing the wall.

- Bend your left knee and grab hold of your left ankle or foot behind you. If you cannot reach it easily use a strap around your foot.

- Lean forward slightly as you take your left leg further behind you.

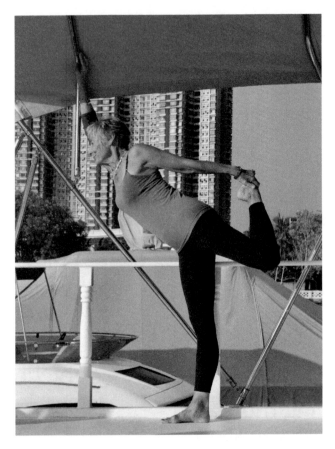

- Hold this pose for 5 breaths before changing sides.

The wall comes in very handy in this balance pose. We are using a pole to hold
onto again in the photo which works just
as well. If you feel this stretch in your

left knee then release it. Push your foot into your hand strongly and try to open out the back of your knee more. This pose also gives a slight backbend to your spine which is energizing.

See a video of the Wall Dancer Pose by scanning the QR code below or at the following link: https://youtu.be/BA1YXT EuxgQ

Wall Warrior 1

- Stand with the right side of your

body close to the wall.

- Step your right foot forward and your left leg back.

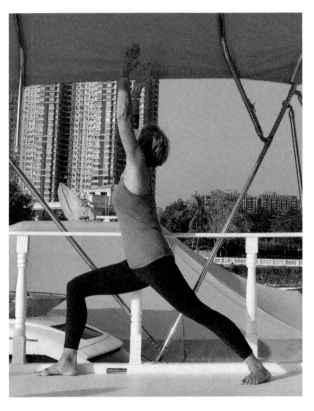

- Bend your right knee at a 90-degree angle and turn your back foot out to a diagonal. Your right hip, knee, and shoulder will be in contact with the wall.

- Keep your back leg straight and your hips facing your front knee.

- Lift your arms overhead and gaze slightly upwards to make a gentle curve with your whole spine.

- Hold this pose for 5 breaths before changing sides.

Once again we are using a railing in place of a wall. This Warrior 1 pose builds up your strength. The wall helps with balance and stability.

See a video of the Wall Warrior 1 by scanning the QR code below or at the following link: https://youtu.be/z761nEUzuR4

Get a FREE PDF download of the Challenging Wall Poses by scanning the QR code below or at the link: https://dl.bookfunnel.com/ctvgl04187

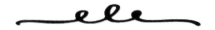

Chapter 5

Partner Poses

Poses with a friend or family member are such fun. You will most likely find yourselves really laughing together. Practicing yoga alongside a trusted partner takes you to a beautiful space where connection and support intertwine.

Partner yoga for couples fosters a unique sense of togetherness, **deepening the bond between partners**. As you embark on this journey together, trust, communication, and teamwork become essential. By working in tandem, you learn to rely on each other's strength and stability, ultimately creating a stronger connection both on and off the mat.

One of the exceptional benefits of partner yoga is the opportunity to enhance **physical alignment.** Practicing alongside a partner allows you to help each other align your bodies, ensuring safer and more effective poses. The added support from a partner allows for a deeper, more fulfilling stretch, enabling a greater range of motion and flexibility.

Partner yoga helps to unlock flexibility and achieve **deeper stretching**. By integrating certain poses that require the support of a partner, you can experience a more profound stretch that would be challenging to achieve on your own. As you work together, you can gently guide and encourage each other to expand your boundaries and explore new realms of flexibility.

Partner yoga encourages **heightened body awareness**, both in oneself and your partner. By connecting and coordinating movements, you become more attuned to your body's sensations and limitations. This awareness allows for a more mindful practice, leading to improved body control, balance, and posture.

Here are some partner yoga poses to try:

Partner Warrior 1

- Stand facing each other with the

toes of one foot touching.

- Step the other leg back turning the foot out to 45 degrees, mirroring each other.

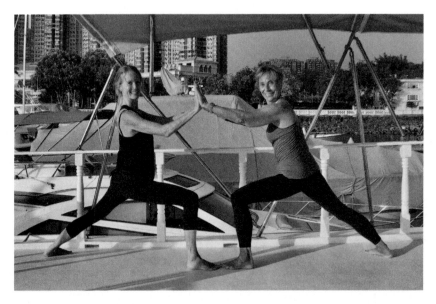

- Bend your front leg at 90 degrees and keep your back leg straight.

- Press your palms together and bring your chests back until your shoulders are above your hips.

- Stay here for 5 breaths before changing sides.

Partner Gate Pose

- Kneel next to each other on a mat.

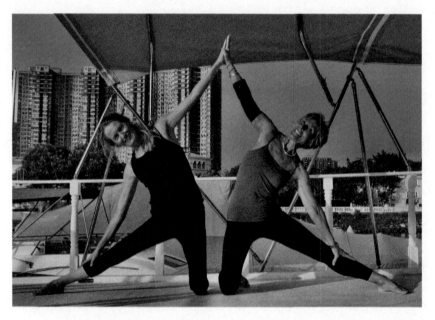

- Put your outer legs straight out to the sides with your toes pointing out to the sides.

- Reach down over your straight

leg, placing your hands below your knees if possible.

- Lift your arms that are closest to each other placing your palms into each other for balance.

- Hold the pose for 5 breaths before changing sides.

This pose provides a strong stretch to your waist. Try not to hold your breath.

Partner Boat Pose

- Sit facing your partner

- Lift your legs and place the soles of your feet against your partners.

- Hold each other's hands here and balance on your sitting bones.

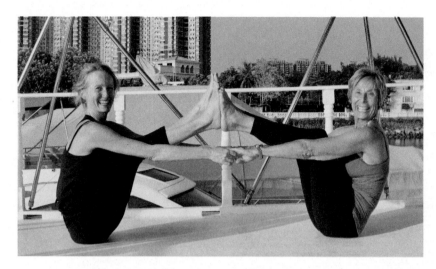

- Stay in this boat pose for up to 5 breaths. Repeat if you can. It is a challenging one!

The **shared laughter and joy** that partner yoga brings adds elements of playfulness and spontaneity to your yoga practice.

As you explore new poses together, you may stumble, wobble, and fall. The lightness and enjoyment derived from partner yoga enhance the overall experience and create lasting memories.

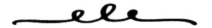

Chapter 6

Pet Protection

There are many health benefits of keeping a pet. In this modern and fast-paced world, where stress and anxiety have become prevalent, finding ways to improve our health and well-being has never been more critical.

One such method that has been gaining recognition as a source of comfort and support is keeping a pet. The benefits that come with owning a pet, extend beyond just companionship. From physical perks to mental and emotional support, the positive impact of having a furry friend in our lives is undeniable.

The main **physical health benefit** of owning a pet is that it encourages a **more active lifestyle**.

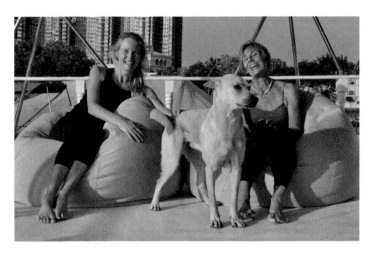

Whether you have a dog that needs regular walks or a cat that loves play-time, pets become our fitness compan-ions. Engaging in physical activities with our pets helps us maintain a healthy body weight and boosts cardiovascular health.

Studies have shown that pet owners tend to have **lower blood pressure and cholesterol levels** than non-pet owners.

The presence of a pet can help reduce stress levels, which in turn contributes to these positive health effects. Stroking their coats and interacting with our furry friends can release endorphins that have a calming effect on our bodies.

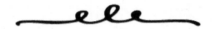

Chapter 7

Can Food Change Your Life

The kinds of foods that have the potential to really kickstart your health are fruits and vegetables.

"A fear of fruit stops far too many people from protecting their health. It mostly stems from the major misconception that the sugar in fruit is the same as refined table sugar and high fructose corn syrup. This is absolutely not the case." Anthony Williams, 2016.

In his #1 New York Times best-seller book, Life-Changing Foods, which has sold millions of copies worldwide, Williams explains that certain fruits, vegetables, herbs, and spices can help us to heal on many levels.

It is interesting to learn about the spiritual lessons of these foods too. Grapes, for instance, help us when we feel isolated because of how they are bunched together on the vine (like a community). Figs help us to make wise choices due to the fact that the fig tree is a landmark of wisdom.

Leafy greens help us to seize opportunities when they arise due to their short shelf life. Potatoes ground us and give us strength because they grow in the ground clustered together like a family. Raw Honey helps good memories stick due to its sticky nature.

Bananas contain fiber, water, potassium, bioavailable protein, and essential omegas.

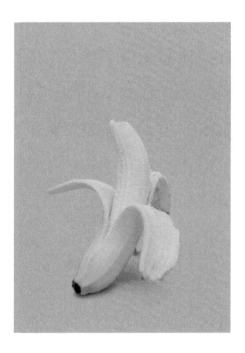

What do you believe about fruit? Have you tried eating it as a morning cleanse?

Eating fruit all morning until lunchtime is a refreshing way to allow your liver to detoxify and give it a rest from eating anything containing overt fats.

Fruit is also ultimately hydrating. Try it, and if you get hungry... You guessed it, eat another piece of fruit.

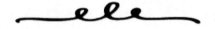

Chapter 8

Find Nourishment

What feeds you other than food? To look at your health from a holistic perspective, think about what makes you feel nourished. Is it the feeling of sea sand underneath your feet?

Perhaps you are more of a water person and being in the water is just what you need for balance. For both my husband and daughter, a swim will wipe out any negativity in their moods – especially if it's in the ocean. You will find them even on a wintery day, surfing or swimming to energize themselves.

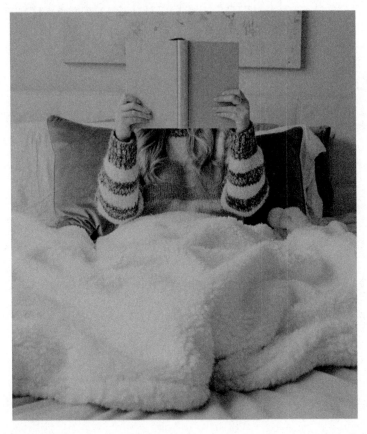

Perhaps you like relaxing in a hot bath or curling up with a book on the sofa. Remind yourself of these things when you feel as if you need a reward of some sort.

Too often we think it's a treat to sit with our phones or to binge on Netflix however these activities usually do not nourish us as well as some of the other more wholesome ones do. Here are some examples:

-Dance to your favourite song, or put a Zumba playlist from YouTube on and dance along.

-Bake a cake or make a healthy no-bake slice (see recipe below for no-bake carrot cake).

-Make your favourite hot drink and sit for a moment savouring it and just allowing your mind to daydream.

-Plan your next holiday. Exploring places to visit and having something to look forward to are motivating.

-Look at old photos. This is guaranteed to bring a smile to your face and a warm feeling to your heart.

-Write someone a letter. A real hand-written letter is a gem. Receiving something by post (other than bills) is an uplifting experience.

-Walk in a garden, city park or beach. Anywhere you can find in your area that has a few trees and some birds. Listen to the birds and give thanks to nature for being there even if you are in a built-up area.

-Plan a date with your partner or an outing with a friend. This also gives you both something to look forward to and strengthens your relationships.

-Take a look at the books on your book-shelf. Are there any that you have been meaning to read? Any you would like to donate to free up some space? Start reading that classic you've always meant to read. I am always amazed at how rele-vant books written sometimes 100 years ago are to today.

-Declutter your closet. This seems like a lot of work, however, the feeling of light-ness and clarity you get afterwards is well worth the effort. If you have clothes that do not fit you anymore or some-thing you haven't worn in over a year, it's often a relief to let them go.

-Attend a class you have always wanted to. Perhaps it's vinyasa Yoga, art, Span-ish or cooking that interests you. Stimulating your brain keeps you young and feeling vibrant.

Make a list of your own so that next time you are feeling out of sorts you can choose something to raise your vibration.

Do it in your own time so it's not overwhelming!

Recipe for No-Bake Carrot Cake:

1.5 cups grated carrot

1.5 cups soaked pitted dates

1.5 cups walnuts

1/2 cup almond meal

1 teaspoon cinnamon

1 teaspoon vanilla essence

1/2 teaspoon ginger

Pinch nutmeg

Pinch cardamom

2 Tablespoons chopped almonds or walnuts for topping

Topping:

1 cup cashews

200 ml coconut cream

Juice of one lemon

1 Tablespoon maple syrup

1/2 teaspoon vanilla essence

Pinch salt

Directions:

Place walnuts into a high-speed blender or food processor and pulse until roughly chopped. Do not make it too fine as you want to keep some texture. Remove the nuts and place them into a mixing bowl. Place dates into a high-speed blender or food processor and blend until fairly smooth. Add this to your mixing bowl with the carrots, spices, vanilla essence and almond meal. Mix until well combined. Press this dough-like mixture into a glass or metal square dish. Place it in the freezer.

To make the topping, add all topping ingredients to a high-speed blender until smooth. Pour this over the carrot cake base and top with the chopped nuts. Place this back in the freezer for an hour or two before you take it out and slice it. Enjoy this healthy and delicious slice with a cup of herbal tea.

See recommendations for fragrant **herbal teas** on my website: https://me lindawright72.wixsite.com/website

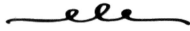

Chapter 9

The Journey Continues

Throughout these pages, we have delved into a myriad of wall yoga exercises, exploring the endless possibilities that arise when we blend the power of the wall with the wisdom of yoga.

In this concluding chapter, I invite you to reflect on how you may initially have felt trepidation when facing the wall, unsure of what it could offer you. As you persevered you may have discovered that the wall is your ally, supporting you, challenging you, and ultimately transforming you.

Take a moment to appreciate what you have achieved. Notice how your body has become **stronger, more flexible, and more resilient**. Subtle shifts within your mind and spirit may also be detected. You have cultivated a newfound sense of balance, both on and off the mat.

Wall Yoga is not just about physical postures; it is a gateway to self-discovery, self-love, and transformation.

As you step away from this book, carry the lessons you have learned with you. Allow the wisdom of the wall to seep into every aspect of your life, reminding you to find strength in the face of challenges, to lean into support when needed, and to trust in your own ability to thrive.

Thank you for joining me on this journey of Wall Yoga. May your practice continue to evolve and deepen, both on and off the mat.

Namaste.

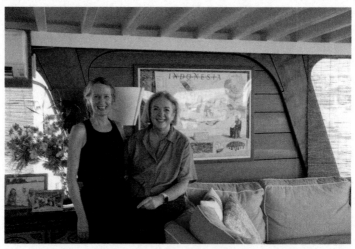

Joan (photographer) and I

Please enjoy your FREE Chair Yoga Bonus book coming up next.

Chapter 10

About our Model

Sytske Kimman is the lovely lady you see in the photos. She has been regularly attending Yoga and Pilates lessons with me for the last 12 years. She is also an avid sailor and loves the ocean, the beach, and the outdoors in general.

Sytske also keeps active hiking. Unfortunately, she has recently been diagnosed with Leukemia. You may have noticed the band on her arm in all the photos which is covering a port for her chemotherapy. Sytske is doing as well as she can. She is both physically and mentally strong.

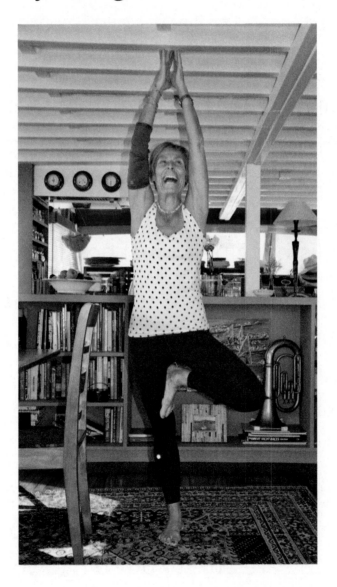

She has already undergone 5 chemotherapy rounds where she needs to go to the hospital for a week at a time.

Sytske does her Yoga and Pilates classes online from her Ward at the hospital when she is there. The doctors and nurses encourage this and they wait for her to finish her class sometimes before administering her drip if possible.

Send out your love to her as she undergoes her biggest challenge yet when she will be required to be in an isolation ward for 5 weeks (October/ November 2023).

This reminds us all how precious and sometimes fragile our health can be. Do what you are able to do so that you can invest in your health. I always imagine health like a bank account. When you do good things for your health, like exercising and eating well, you put money in your health bank account. When your activities include "bad" things like drinking too much coffee and alcohol, eating fatty foods, missing your workouts and allowing stress to govern your life, then you are taking money out of your health bank account.

Make sure your health bank account is looking abundant and then if you do experience any setbacks, like Sytske, you can deal with them all the better.

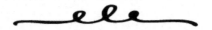

About the Author

Melinda Wright is a certified group exercise instructor, Personal Trainer, and Yoga and Pilates teacher. She specializes in working with people of all levels of fitness to provide safe and effective exercise sessions for them. She has developed ways of using Yoga, Pilates, and strength training to improve the well-being of her clients and help them to become healthier as they age. She makes it easy to learn any Yoga and Pilates exercise as she is encouraging and patient, using easy-to-understand explanations.

She helps people to feel good about themselves and their exercise sessions.

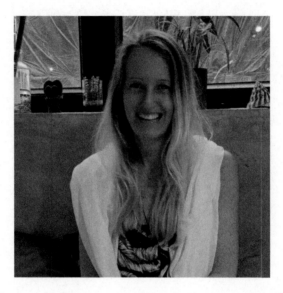

Melinda's life purpose is to help people of all ages learn and practice Yoga and Pilates regardless of any physical limitations they may have. She also instills in them a passion for these disciplines increasing their body-mind connection and leaving them feeling flexible, younger, and more energized.

Melinda has worked worldwide (South Africa, New Zealand, the United Kingdom, Hong Kong, and Australia) in health and fitness for more than 30 years.

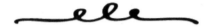

Also By

https://a.co/d/aiSS47O

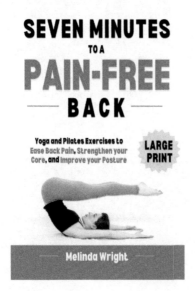

https://a.co/d/7qJucHp

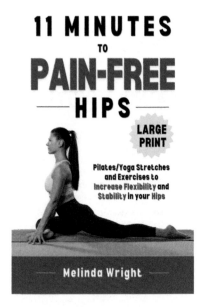

https://a.co/d/92rmQbU

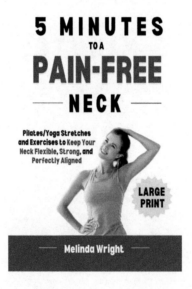

https://a.co/d/9sziopC

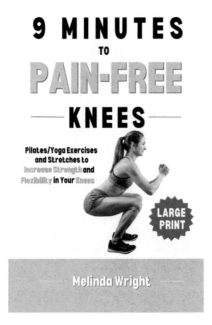

https://a.co/d/iQpCqJ6

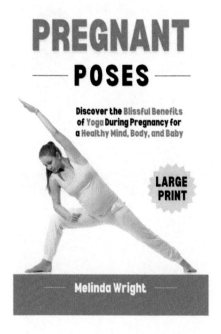

https://a.co/d/07TpMrV

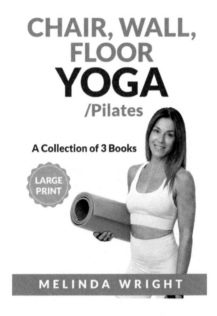

CHAIR, WALL,
FLOOR
YOGA
/Pilates

A Collection of 3 Books

LARGE
PRINT

MELINDA WRIGHT

Acknowledgements

I am truly grateful to the following individuals who have provided me with help and support. Without them, this book would not be here.

Pauline Ching, my friend, editor, and accountability partner who checks in with me regularly.

Joan Bouttell, who selflessly takes time out of her busy life to take amazing photos and makes the sessions fun.

Our gorgeous model, Sytske Kimman, for making the poses look so good.

Tracey Godfrey for graciously providing her copyrighting skills.

Caroline Oliver, for your support and input. The world needs more compassionate doctors like you who are a good example of health and vitality.

Robyn Haddican, Emma Place, Sarah Fairhurst, Bart Kimman, and Diana Marchenko, who are regular clients in the studio, inspire me to keep daily classes running.

All my other clients, who have supported me throughout the years.

My friends, Kasia Stawiarska, Ralitsa Ivanova, Pebble Loh, and many more who support me.

The Medical Medium, for speaking the truth about healing and helping so many people who suffer from chronic illnesses.

My angels and guides, who lead me every day.

Mom and Dad, for all your love and support from afar.

My loving and supportive husband, Greg.

My beautiful daughter, Amy for being true to yourself and giving my life meaning.

I am truly grateful to you all. I appreciate all you add to my life!

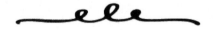

CHAIR YOGA

Yoga for Seniors, Beginners and Office Workers for Strength, Flexibility and Balance

LARGE PRINT

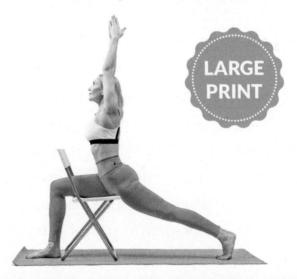

MELINDA WRIGHT

reading this document, the reader agrees that under no circumstances is the author responsible for any losses, direct or indirect, which are incurred as a result of the use of the information contained within this document, including, but not limited to, errors, omissions, or inaccuracies.

Contents

Foreword

I strongly recommend this book "Chair Yoga" for anyone who is starting yoga, or perhaps is a senior with less confidence in the practice. As with her other books, she gives very pragmatic advice on which are the best exercises to do, in this case, with a chair. There are clear and concise instructions with clear photos for each exercise. The videos via a QR code are also very helpful.

Melinda is a wonderful Yoga and Pilates instructor who uses her wealth of experience to explain the most effective methods of approaching yoga practice. I have been very fortunate to have been able to attend her classes regularly for years and know firsthand how successful her methods are. Her warm and engaging style really motivates you whether in person or via the book.

As a GP, I am increasingly seeing patients with symptoms associated with lack of exercise or poor nutrition. I feel we would all benefit from following Melinda's advice and exercises.

Thank you, Melinda, for writing such an excellent helpful book, guiding us to improve our well-being! Also many thanks to Sytske for being such an inspiring model despite her current circum-

stances, and to Joan the skilled photographer.

Caroline Oliver

MBBS FRCGP

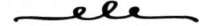

Chapter 1

Why Use a Chair?

Grab a seat! In this book, we will explore the benefits of practicing Yoga and Pilates exercises while sitting.

Whether you are recovering from an injury, spend a lot of time sitting at work, or if you are a senior citizen, then this book will teach you how to improve your health and well-being from the comfort of your chair.

You will discover how these exercises can improve **strength, flexibility,** and

posture, as well as reduce stress and increase relaxation.

With easy-to-follow instructions and clear photos, you'll be able to begin your Chair Yoga and Pilates practice right away.

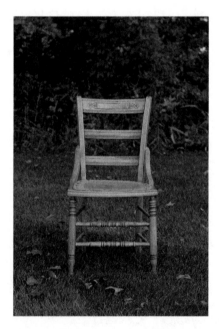

There are also links via **QR codes** to take you straight to videos showing you exactly how to do these chair exercises. So, sit back, relax, and get ready to feel the benefits of this transformative practice.

Just because you are in a chair doesn't mean that you cannot work every muscle, joint, ligament, and tendon in your body. Chair Yoga can gently and gradually bring you to a higher state of physical and mental fitness while helping you to feel relaxed and safe at the same time.

Yoga means a union between the mind, body, and spirit, and they are all connected through our breathing. "The medical applications of Yoga are numerous: It can help those with heart disease, high blood pressure, musculoskeletal problems, and in particular with the prevention and treatment of back pain." (Pullig Schatz MD, 2016).

The exercises in this book are mainly traditional Yoga poses modified in order to be performed on a chair for support. In some cases the chair makes us work even harder and go deeper into certain poses as we feel confident with the additional support it provides.

You will learn some easy exercises that you can do anywhere there is a chair or even a bench.

You may be surprised at how effective these **exercises and stretches** are as they are relaxing and easy to do.

Perhaps you chose Chair Yoga because you are in pain or you are immobile in some way. It's challenging to do anything at all when you are suffering, let alone find the motivation to exercise.

Please listen to your body and check with your doctor if it's suitable for you to begin an exercise regime.

You will benefit from my decades of experience as a Yoga and Pilates instructor, group exercise teacher, and personal trainer. I have been helping people to keep their bodies strong and flexible for over 30 years.

This book is short, easy to read, and designed for any level of fitness or age. I will get straight into the exercises soon so you can get results as quickly as possible.

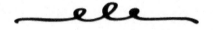

Chapter 2

Let's Move!

Exercise is without a doubt one of the most crucial elements of keeping a healthy lifestyle. Regular exercise keeps your body physically fit, and it also has numerous benefits for your mental and emotional well-being. In this chapter, we'll explore the importance of exercise and how it can positively impact all aspects of your life.

First and foremost, exercise is essential for maintaining a **healthy body weight.** When you engage in physical activity, your body burns calories and uses energy, which helps to prevent the accumulation of excess body fat. This, in turn, reduces the risk of obesity, heart disease, and other chronic health conditions.

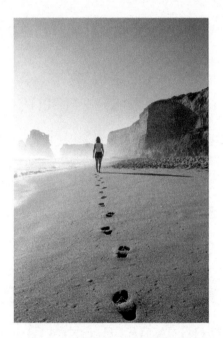

Exercise is a crucial component of **building and maintaining healthy bones, muscles, and joints.** When you engage in weight-bearing exercises, your bones, and muscles are subjected to small amounts of stress, which stimulates their growth and strength. This can reduce the risk of osteoporosis and other bone-related conditions.

Additionally, exercise is critical for improving **cardiovascular health**. When you exercise, your heart rate increases, which helps to strengthen the heart muscle and improve blood flow. This, in turn, lowers your risk of developing high blood pressure, heart disease, and the incidence of strokes.

Mental and emotional well-being is another area where exercise can have a significant impact. Exercise has been shown to reduce stress, anxiety, and depression by reducing levels of cortisol and increasing the production of endorphins, known as the "feel-good" hor-mones. This can help to boost self-es-teem, improve mood, and promote overall mental and emotional well-be-ing.

Finally, exercise is critical for maintain-ing a **high level of energy** and improv-ing overall quality of life. Regular exer-cise has been shown to increase ener-gy levels, reduce fatigue, and improve sleep quality. This can help to keep you feeling great and performing at your best in all aspects of your life.

If you fail to exercise you may experi-ence either of the following:

Tight muscles

Muscles may become shortened and thus feel tight due to either too much activity or too little. If there is a continuous, repetitive movement that you perform every day in your daily life, this could cause pain and tightness in the muscles. Sitting in a certain position for too long may also cause these muscles to tighten. Also, standing too long may cause your muscles to become fatigued and prone to spasms. Lack of stretching also causes muscles to shorten and feel tight.

Weak muscles

Our muscles need to be strong to hold us upright all day and to perform our daily tasks. They may become fatigued causing pain and stiffness if they are not worked regularly. Weak muscles also contribute to a lack of energy and fatigue.

As you can see, exercise is a critical component of maintaining a healthy lifestyle. It offers numerous physical, mental, and emotional benefits that can positively impact your overall well-being.

Whether you're an older adult or a younger beginner, it's never too late to start incorporating exercise into your daily routine.

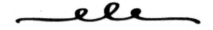

Chapter 3

Ready to Start?

These simple chair exercises and stretches will bring blood flow to your muscles and joints and thus aid in your fitness, strength, and healing. Stretching also nurtures your joints by slowing down the degeneration that occurs with aging.

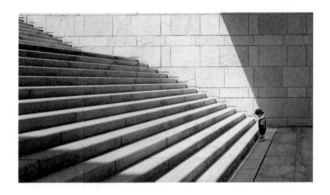

What you will need is a **sturdy chair** on a flat non-slip surface.

Clothing

Wear comfortable clothing that makes it easy for you to move in. Your clothing should not be too baggy as it gets in the way, and not too tight, as this restricts movement. You are welcome to be barefoot however if you prefer to wear shoes make sure that they allow you to move freely and are not too bulky. If you wear socks make sure they have a grip on the bottom so that you do not slip.

Hydration

Make sure you are well hydrated by drinking a glass of water or juice. Keep a water bottle handy so that if you become thirsty during your workout you can easily reach it. Do not work out on a full stomach. If you do need to eat something right before exercising fruit is perfect as it is very easy to digest and provides you with instant energy.

Surface

It is preferable for you to use a non-slip mat. For a recommendation of my favorite mat scan the QR code below or visit the following link: https://melindawright72.wixsite.com/website

Connect with your Body

This is best done via your breathing. As soon as you bring your awareness to your breathing, a natural link between your mind and body is established.

If you cannot breathe during an exercise you are working too hard. Ease off a little and take a deep breath before continuing. Notice how your body is feeling and stand up tall with good posture.

Check in with your body regularly throughout your workout being sure not to overexert yourself or work through any pain. If you do feel pain, stop and assess it. Undue stress on the body can lead to fatigue so exercise within your limits and build yourself up slowly.

Be Patient

It takes time to get the results you may be hoping for. They definitely do not arrive overnight.

Yoga is a highly effective way to improve your overall well-being and fitness however requires a commitment to doing the exercises consistently. Even 10 or 20 minutes is enough at first and you will soon be able to enjoy the benefits that come from a regular practice.

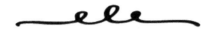

Chapter 4

Seated Chair Exercises

Chair Hip Stretch

Use a chair, bench, or even a stool for this exercise.

- Sit down and cross your right leg over your left leg.

- Circle your foot around your ankle a few times in one direction, then in the other direction. Flex your foot and hold it as though you are wearing a boot.

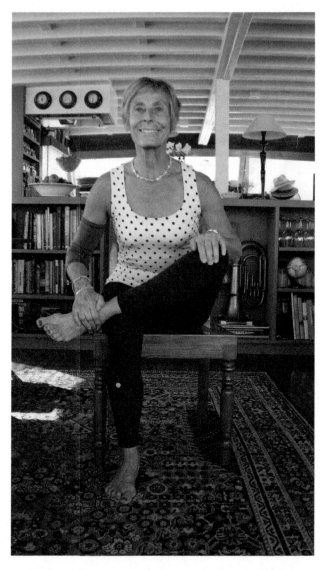

- Keep your back as straight as possible and gently push your knee down and out to the side. Your knee may not want to move down much.

Just do what you can, remembering not to move through any pain.

- Breathe deeply as you bring your chest forward a couple of centimeters. Keep your back fairly straight. Let your chest lead the way rather than rounding your back.

- Push your knee down as far as it will go and remember to breathe deeply for about 3 to 5 breaths.

You will usually feel a stretching sensation in the hip area. This simple hip opener stretches the glute muscles.

If you have relatively tight hips your knee will be a bit higher up than shown in the photo. You are still getting a good hip stretch wherever your knee may be. You will still feel the stretch in the right place which is in the glutes.

Remember to flex your foot as this keeps the ankle straight and prevents overstretching on the outside of the ankle.

If you feel this in your knees find a way to bring the stretch into your gluteus muscles.

You may need to straighten the bottom leg out if your top leg is unable to get on top of the other one easily. Be patient with your body – it's doing its best!

See a video of the **Chair Hip Stretch** by scanning the QR code below or at the link: https://youtu.be/PgdhGowMte0

Chair Warrior 2

- Sit on a sturdy chair. Slide your right leg off the right side of the chair, keeping your right buttock fully supported by the seat.

- Position yourself so that your back leg is off the left side of the chair and is not supported much at all.

If necessary you may need to use a yoga block underneath your right foot if the chair is too high.

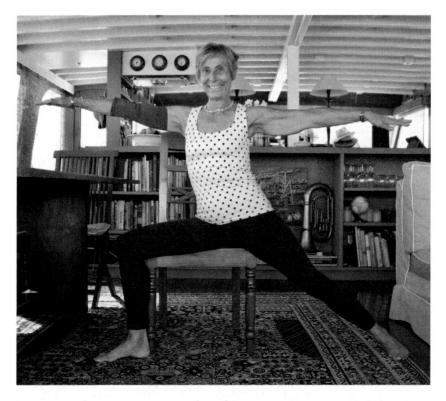

Try to keep good alignment with your front leg bent at 90 degrees and your back leg straight. Keep your hips facing forwards with your shoulders directly above your hips.

- Take your arms up and out to the sides. Keep your arms strong and straight. Press your feet into the floor, almost as if the chair is not there, and imagine doing this pose free-standing.

- Take 3 to 5 breaths here. You can choose to look over your right arm and set an intention with your mind.

See a video of Chair Warrior 2 by scanning the QR code below or at the following link: https://youtube.com/shorts/lqE_fReRP3w?feature=share

Chair Side Angle

- Sit on a sturdy chair. Slide your right leg off the right side of the chair, keeping your right buttock fully supported by the seat.

- Position yourself so that your back leg is off the left side of the chair and is not supported much at all.

- Place your right elbow onto your inner right knee and extend your

left arm over your head. Try to extend into a diagonal line with the
left side of your body.

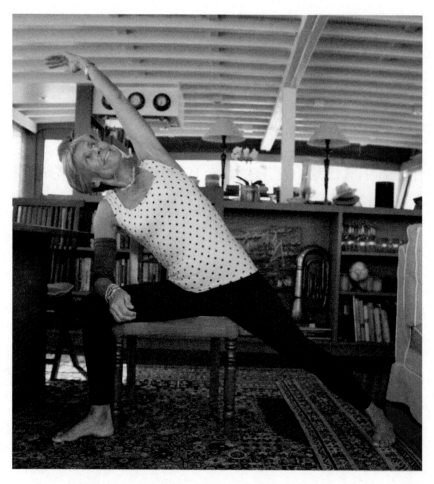

- Look up towards the ceiling on the
  inside of your arm and keep your

neck in a straight line with your spine.

- Take about 5 breaths here before changing sides.

This pose stretches your waist and strengthens your legs.

Press into your feet and pretend that the chair is not there to challenge yourself.

See a video of the Chair Side Angle Pose by scanning the QR code or at the following link: https://youtube.com/shorts/xQDeOuvCVbA?feature=share

Chair Quad Stretch

- Sit on a sturdy chair and turn to the right side.

- Hold on to the backrest of the chair to keep you balanced.

- Bend your left knee and grab your left ankle or foot. If you are unable to reach your foot use a strap around it. Point your left knee down to the floor and keep your hips under your shoulders.

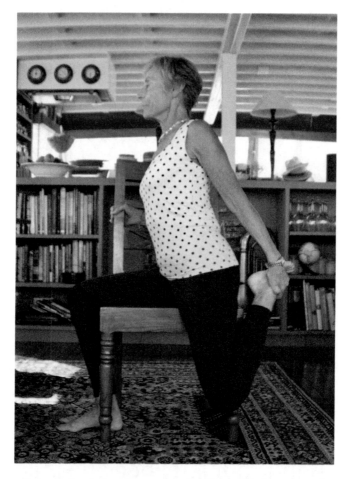

- Hold this stretch for 5 breaths and then change sides.

You can look forward and lift your chest to ensure good posture. To increase the stretch bring your heel closer to your left buttock and also tilt your pelvis underneath you a little so that you are not arching your back. Keep your navel pulled in towards your spine.

See a video of the Seated Quad Stretch by scanning the QR code below or at the following link: https://youtube.com/shorts/A8YV2qYMcyl?feature=share

Chair Backbend

- Sit slightly forward on the chair.

- Grip the sides of the seat as you lean back and curve into a backend. Lift your chest as well so that the backbend is felt in the middle and upper back and also your neck.

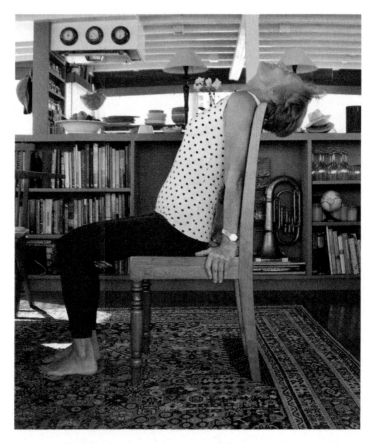

- Take 3 breaths here.

You may need to shift your position depending on the chair you are using to make it more comfortable.

Backbends are fantastic for our posture because most of our activities in daily life cause us to lean forward and sometimes even slouch.

Poses like this counteract forward stooping posture and open the chest and shoulder muscles.

See a video on the Chair Backbend by scanning the QR code below or at the following link: https://youtube.com/shorts/mdDL7kWRIn0?feature=share

Chair Twist

- Sit sideways on your sturdy chair.

- Keep your feet flat on the floor and your sitting bones evenly pressing down into the seat of the chair.

- Turn towards the backrest of the chair and pull yourself around into a twist.

- Hold this twist for 3 to 5 breaths before changing sides.

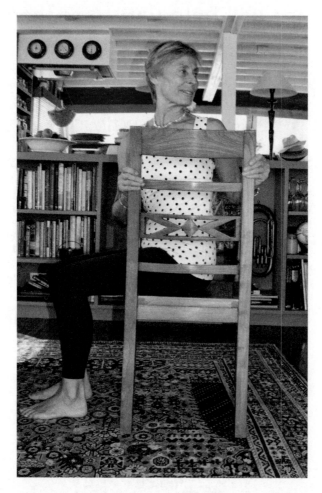

Keep your spine long and straight while you are twisting. Imagine that it is an axis and twist around it.

Your breathing may be a little shallower in your twist.

This pose will help you to realign your spine and release tension in your back muscles. Twists also help to trim the waistline and to detoxify our internal organs.

See a video on the Chair Twist by scanning the QR code below or at the following link: https://youtube.com/shorts/YcA2Z785KJM?si=3oEyBZnbCNfQdkZd

Get your free PDF Quick Reference Guide for all the Seated Chair Exercises by scanning the QR code below or at the following link: https://dl.bookfunnel.com/fg9raripdf

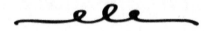

Chapter 5

Standing Chair Exercises

Chair Calf Raises

- Stand behind the chair with the backrest facing you.

- Hold onto the backrest of the chair. **Lift and lower** your heels from the floor as you keep your legs straight. Press all of your toes evenly into the floor. Lift up as high as you can so that you feel this in the calf muscles.

- Do **15 to 30 repetitions** until your calf muscles begin to burn a little.

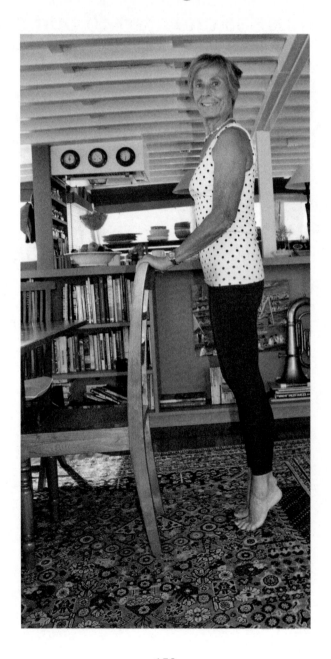

This is a great exercise for better circulation. Our calf muscles act like mini heart muscles and start to pump more blood around the body. If you work in an office, are on a long flight, or are stuck inside during bad weather, this is a great exercise to keep your blood flowing and improve your circulation!

See a video of Standing Calf Raises by scanning the QR code below or at the following link: https://youtube.com/shorts/LxkFdY19ZBc?feature=share

Chair L-shape

- Stand behind the chair holding the backrest.

- Walk your feet away until they are underneath your hips and make a table-top shape with your back.

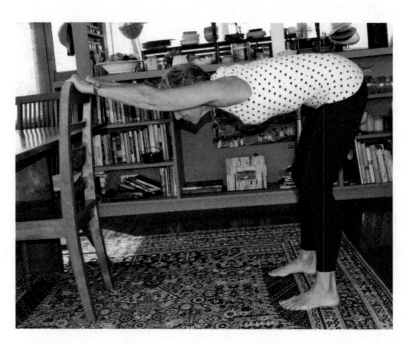

- Keep your ears in line with your

arms and tuck your chin looking down to the floor.

- Take 5 breaths here before coming up.

If you find that your back is rounded bend your knees and drive your hips back and try to keep your back as straight as possible.

It's best to do this Chair L–shape stretch 3 times. You will most likely find that by your third one, your back is at its straightest.

It gives a satisfying stretch to the muscles on either side of the spine and relieves back spasms and backache.

See a video of Chair L-Shape by scanning the QR code below or at the following link: https://youtu.be/dnb0BpHBBxk

Chair Tree Pose

- Stand strong and straight with your feet slightly apart. Draw an imaginary line up through the center of your body.

- Lift your right leg up and place the sole of your right foot on the inner side of your left leg. You may choose to place it down closer to the ankle or even rest the toes on the floor. Make sure that your right foot is not pushing into the side of the left knee. Place the sole of your foot either above or below your knee.

- Keep your gaze steady on one spot. Choose something close by that is not moving at first and then challenge yourself to look further away. Imagine that you are a tree with roots growing out of your foot deep into the center of the earth.

- Hold the tree pose for about 5 breaths or longer and then

change sides.

Visualize your root system being strong and stable.

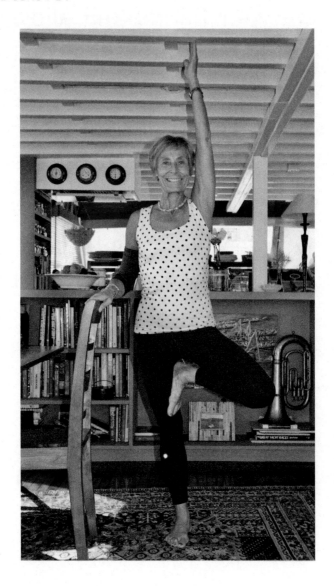

Once you have your balance you may like to take your arms over your head.

Keep your hands together at first then separate your hands and allow your arms to fall out to the sides with the palms of your hands facing up. Soften your arms here and feel like you are in a receiving mode. Be open to all the good that can come your way.

Healthy trees are supple and move gently in the wind. If you hold your body too rigidly here you will feel like your energy is stuck and you may feel brittle.

Let yourself go and remember to laugh at yourself if you wobble in your tree pose. We all have some days that we balance better than others.

Performing this tree pose near a wall or chair helps you to balance and keeps you safe from falling. Release all self-judgment and try again on the other side. Try to hold the tree pose for a minute or more on each side.

This pose is good for the legs as it strengthens your feet and ankles, using all your proprioceptive muscles for balance.

Tree pose encourages synchronicity between the right and left hemispheres of your brain.

Chair Triangle

- Stand next to the seat of the chair. Open your legs out with your right foot under the seat of the chair. If you measured the length of one of your legs, then the distance between your feet should be that far apart.

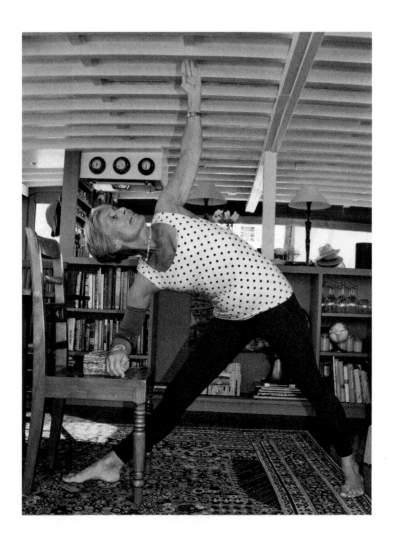

- Turn your right foot out to the right side and your left foot inwards about 5 centimeters. Square your hips to the front. Imagine that you are holding a bowl of water in your pelvis.

- Tip your hips to the right and pretend that you are pouring this water out through a spout down your right leg. This deepens the crease at the top of the right leg where it meets the torso and lengthens both sides of the waist.

- Keep both legs straight and strong, and press all four corners (your big toe, your little toe, your outer heel, and your inner heel) of both feet into the mat. Extend your arm down to the chair and place your palm or elbow on the chair. You may use a brick to make it the correct height for you.

- Place your top hand on your hip. Make sure that you are leaning directly over your right leg and try to prevent your hips from going to the back and your chest from going forward.

- When you feel open in your chest lift your top arm straight up to the sky in line with your bottom arm.

- Look either down, forward, or up, depending on how your neck feels. Keep your spine long and straight. Smile and enjoy the expansive feeling in the hips and heart with this triangle pose. Stay in this pose for 3 to 5 breaths.

You may choose to keep your left hand on your hip if you feel tired.

The chair helps you to balance.

Scan the QR code below to see a video of the Triangle Pose or visit the link: https://youtu.be/2BsjUI3HUp4

<u>Chair Forward Bend</u>

- Stand in front of the chair facing the seat.

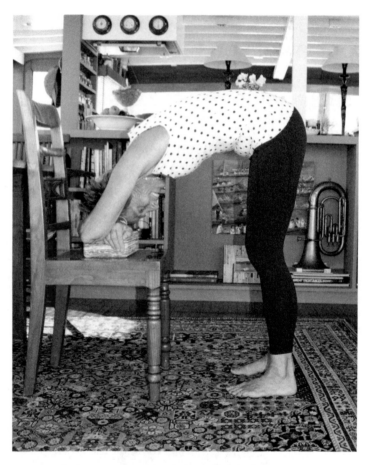

- Fold at your hip creases (where your legs meet your torso) and place your hands or your elbows on the chair.

- Keep your hips in line with your heels. Rest over the chair like this using a yoga brick if you need more height.

- Stay here for 5 breaths or more.

Forward bends are generally cooling and calming.

Do you feel good here? If not come up to standing.

Some days forward bends don't feel as comfortable as other days, especially if you have any congestion in your head. Always listen to your body.

Download your FREE PDF Quick Reference Guide for the Standing Chair Exercises by scanning the QR code below or at the following link: https://dl.bookfun nel.com/thoqqml3y9

Chapter 6

Hyperbolic Walking and Rebounding

Rebounding, also known as trampoline exercise, is a fun and effective way to improve your overall well-being. Get ready to bounce your way to better health!

Rebounding has been around for centuries, with its roots dating back to ancient civilizations. It gained popularity in the modern world during the 1930s when trampolines were invented. Initially used by astronauts to counteract the effects of zero gravity, rebounding quickly caught on as a form of exercise.

Rebounding involves jumping on a mini-trampoline or rebounder. The unique mechanism of the trampoline absorbs the impact of each jump, reducing stress on your joints. As you bounce, the rhythmic up-and-down motion engages every muscle in your body, providing a full-body workout.

Rebounding encourages your core muscles and large muscle groups to contract and release again. This results in the rhythmic compression of the veins and arteries, which more effectively moves fluids (blood and lymph) through the body and back to the heart. This lightens the heart's load and lowers peripheral **blood pressure.** Rebounding is an excellent **cardiovascular exercise** that gets your heart pumping and increases blood circulation.

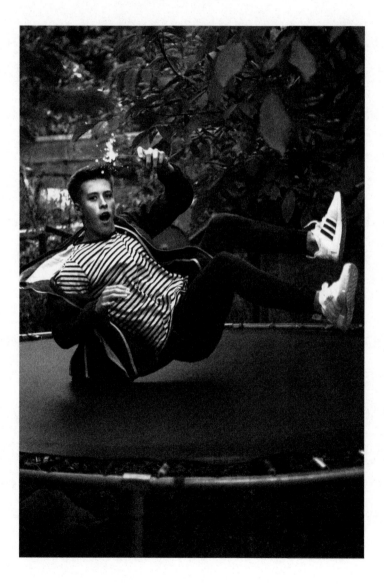

The continuous jumping motion strengthens your heart and improves its efficiency, leading to a healthier cardio-vascular system.

The **lymphatic system** plays a crucial role in removing toxins, waste, and excess fluid from our bodies. Rebounding stimulates lymphatic flow, helping to flush out toxins and boost the immune system. The up-and-down motion acts as a pump, assisting lymphatic fluid circulation throughout the body.

Rebounding engages all of our major muscle groups, including the legs, arms, core, and back. The continuous bouncing motion helps to tone and strengthen these muscles, improving overall **body strength and endurance**. Regular rebounding sessions can lead to leaner and more defined muscles.

Jumping on a trampoline challenges your **balance and coordination**. The controlled movements required for rebounding help improve your body's proprioception, making you more aware of your body's position in space. This can have significant benefits for everyday activities and reduce the risk of falls and injuries.

Rebounding releases feel-good endorphins, reducing stress levels and promoting a **positive mood.** The rhythmic bouncing motion can also have a calming effect, helping to alleviate anxiety and improve overall mental well-being. Regular rebounding sessions can be a great way to destress and unwind after a long day.

Before starting any exercise program, it's essential to take some **safety precautions.** Ensure that your rebounder is in good condition, with no tears or damaged springs. Wear comfortable, athletic shoes to provide proper support and stability. Start with gentle, controlled movements and gradually increase the intensity as your fitness level improves.

There are numerous ways to incorporate rebounding into your fitness routine. You can try simple bouncing, jumping jacks, high knees, or even dance-inspired movements. Mix up your workouts to keep them fun and engaging.

If you do not have access to a rebounder you could try to do what I call hyperbolic walking. It's really just walking with an exaggerated spring in your step almost like you are skipping along (without the extra bounce where your feet leave the floor). You will probably get a few strange looks especially as this kind of walking usually makes you want to sing, hum, or whistle along with it.

This bouncy walking simulates the bouncing that you would do on a mini trampoline.

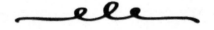

Chapter 7

A Fine Balance

Balance is a skill that can be learned. When astronauts return from a journey in space they walk like they are intoxicated. They need to re-learn how to balance. You can train yourself to improve your balance too. A simple exercise is to stand on one leg. Lift your other leg just off the floor in front of you. Time how long you can stand on one leg without putting your other foot down. Try not to hold onto anything. When this becomes easy, and it will if you practice it, try to do the same thing with your eyes closed.

Don't be disappointed if you cannot hold your balance for more than one second. With practice every day you should even see an improvement in a few days.

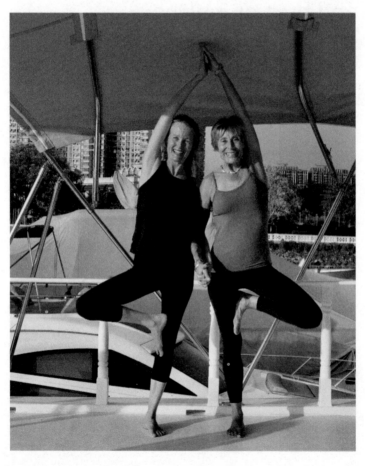

Perhaps you enjoy chair yoga to keep you safe from falling. Balance is a life skill. As we age our balance becomes compromised perhaps due to muscle weakness, vestibular issues, or even viral infections and we are more likely to fall and hurt ourselves.

Enjoy partner Yoga with a friend for added support and fun!

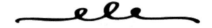

Chapter 8

Please Stand!

"Prolonged sitting (more than 6 hours a day) increases your risk of just about everything, including heart attack, stroke, diabetes, obesity, and cancer". Christiane Northrup (2016)

Sitting is an essential part of modern life. We sit at our desks, in the car, bus, or train, on the couch, and even at the dinner table. The human body is designed to move. Our ancestors spent their days hunting, gathering, and tending to crops. Even just a few decades ago, most jobs required physical labor. However, the advent of technology has led to a drastic reduction in physical activity. Sedentary jobs have become the norm, and most people spend most of their waking hours sitting.

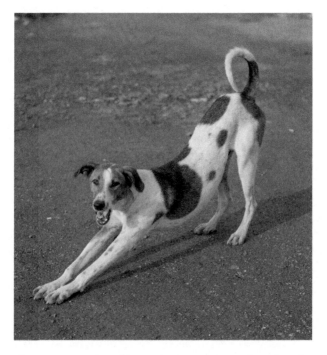

Animals naturally stretch their bodies. Watch your dog or your cat when they wake up and do their stretches.

Research has shown that sitting for extended periods can have a profound impact on our health. A study, conducted by the American Cancer Society, found that women who sit for more than six hours per day are 37% more likely to die prematurely than those who sit for less than three hours.

So, why is sitting so bad for our health? The answer lies in the way our bodies respond to extended periods of inactivity.

When we sit for long periods, our muscles become inactive, leading to a reduction in blood flow. This reduction in blood flow can cause a buildup of fatty acids in our bloodstream, which can lead to obesity, type 2 diabetes, and other metabolic disorders.

Prolonged sitting can also cause our body to burn less fat, leading to an increase in body fat and weight gain. Sitting for long periods can also cause our muscles to weaken, leading to a decrease in muscle mass and strength.

In addition to physical health concerns, prolonged sitting has been linked to mental health issues such as depression and anxiety. Studies have shown that sedentary behavior can lead to increased stress, reduced self-esteem, and even cognitive decline.

Standing for long periods is not the answer either as this also causes strain on the legs and the back muscles. Moving your body regularly is the solution.

To combat these negative health effects of sitting, it's essential to get up and move throughout the day.

Whether it's through regular exercise, taking frequent breaks to stretch and walk, or investing in a standing desk, we must make a conscious effort to reduce prolonged sitting and prioritize physical activity.

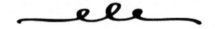

Chapter 9

Connection and Community

There is a healing power of community. In a world where individualism is celebrated, it's easy to overlook the importance of **community and friendship**. There is a profound connection between our social interactions and our overall health. Numerous studies have shown that community and friendship play a vital role in promoting physical, mental, and emotional well-being.

Friendship provides us with an invaluable **support system** that can alleviate stress, anxiety, and depression. When life throws its inevitable challenges at us, having a trusted network to lean on can make all the difference. Sharing our burdens, seeking advice, or simply having someone to talk to can lighten the load and provide us with a sense of emotional well-being. In times of crisis, it is through the strength and compassion of our community that we may find solace and regain our resilience.

When it comes to **maintaining a healthy lifestyle**, the power of community cannot be underestimated. Engaging with like-minded individuals who prioritize their well-being can inspire and motivate us to adopt healthier habits.

Whether it's joining a fitness class, participating in community sports, or cooking nutritious meals together, the contagious enthusiasm and camaraderie of friends can encourage us to make choices that benefit our physical health.

Being a part of a community fosters a **sense of belonging and purpose**, both of which are essential for our overall happiness and well-being. When we feel connected to those around us, we develop a sense of identity and purpose that contributes to our mental and emotional health. Engaging in communal activities, volunteering, or participating in group initiatives gives us a deeper sense of meaning, enabling us to lead more fulfilling lives.

The modern world, with its fast-paced lifestyle and digital connectivity, paradoxically can leave us feeling isolated and lonely. Research has shown that loneliness can have severe impacts on our health, comparable to risk factors such as smoking or obesity. However, by actively cultivating and nurturing friendships and participating in a community, we can combat feelings of isolation and create meaningful connections that fortify our well-being.

Communities offer us the opportunity to access collective wisdom and learn from shared experiences. By engaging with a diverse group of individuals, we open ourselves up to a multitude of perspectives and insights that can help us heal.

According to Brene Brown, #1 New York Times bestselling author, **belonging** is the innate human desire to be part of something larger than ourselves.

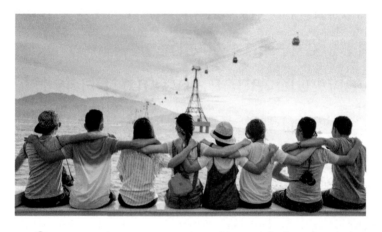

We often try to acquire this by seeking approval and fitting in. However "true belonging only happens when we present our authentic, imperfect selves to the world, our sense of belonging can never be greater than our level of self-acceptance". (Brown, 2017)

If we accept ourselves we will be able to bring our true selves to the party and offer our unique gifts to the whole.

If we are all the same there is nothing new to contribute anyway. Be yourself!

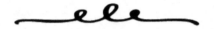

Chapter 10

Relaxation

Your Chair Yoga poses are now complete. It's beneficial to take a little time to relax your body after working on your Chair Yoga Poses. This relaxation is typically done lying flat on the floor however if you are happy to stay seated in your chair you may remain there.

Take a moment to close your eyes and connect with your breath. Feel the steady rhythm of inhalation and exhalation, grounding you in the present moment. Let go of any expectations or judgments you may have about your practice. Instead, focus on cultivating a sense of curiosity and self-compassion.

Start to relax your whole body progressively from your feet upwards. Relax your toes, feet, ankles, calf muscles, knees, and thighs. Moving your attention up to relax your hips, and then your pelvic area, wrapping the relaxation around to your lower back. Move into your belly and feel the rise and fall of the abdomen with your breathing.

You may choose to place your hands on your belly and feel the breath moving the hands. Shift your attention higher up to your upper back and chest. Relax this area as you encourage your mind to stay with your bodily sensations. Take another deep breath into your shoulders and down your arms as you allow your upper arms, elbows, forearms, hands, and fingers to relax.

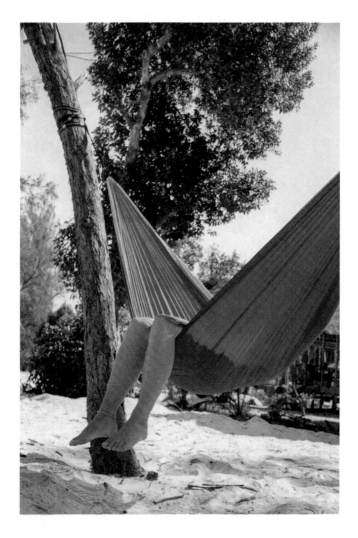

Take your attention back up to your neck and relax the front, sides, and back of the neck. Relax your jaw, face, scalp, and forehead. Scan your body down to your toes again and make sure that the relaxation has reached everywhere. If you find it difficult to let go of tension in certain areas of your body just try to breathe into them.

Now, move your attention to your breathing and let it be as natural as possible, not trying to control the breath at all. Stay here for a few more minutes. Your mind will wander off as it is natural for it to do so.

Gently bring your awareness back to your breathing and your body, giving yourself full permission to relax.

After a few minutes, bring your awareness back to your surroundings and
open your eyes. Roll over onto your right
side (if you were lying down) and move
into a sitting position. Bring your hands
to your sternum and breathe into the
center of your heart.

Namaste

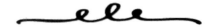

Chapter 11

Embracing the Journey

Throughout these pages, we have explored the art of Chair Yoga and discovered its transformative power. We have learned that Yoga is not just about physical postures; it is a practice that encompasses the mind, body, and spirit.

In this concluding chapter, I would like to invite you to embrace the journey you have embarked upon. Yoga is not a destination, but a lifelong path of self-discovery and growth. It is a practice that evolves with us, adapting to our changing bodies and circumstances.

As you continue on your Chair Yoga journey, remember to be gentle with yourself. There will be days when you feel strong and flexible, and there will be days when you feel tired or stiff. Embrace both the highs and the lows, for they are all part of the beautiful tapestry of life.

As you move through the Chair Yoga exercises and poses, allow your body to guide you. Listen to its wisdom and honor its limitations. Remember that Yoga is not about achieving the perfect pose; it is about finding harmony and balance within yourself.

Beyond the physical benefits, Chair Yoga offers a space for introspection and self-reflection. It is an opportunity to cultivate mindfulness and cultivate a deeper connection with your inner self. Take time to explore the sensations in your body, the thoughts in your mind, and the emotions in your heart.

Find moments of stillness amidst the chaos, breathe deeply when faced with challenges, and practice gratitude for the simple joys that surround you. Allow the lessons you have learned on the mat to permeate every aspect of your existence.

Remember that Yoga is not confined to a specific space or time. You can practice Chair Yoga wherever you are, whether it's at home, at work, or even while traveling. Let your practice become a constant companion, supporting you through the ups and downs of life.

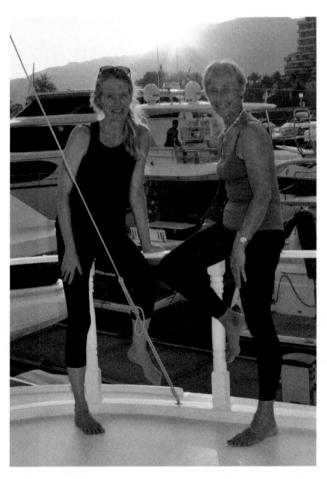

Finally, I encourage you to share your newfound knowledge and love for Chair

Yoga with others. Spread the joy and benefits of this practice to those who may not have access to traditional Yoga classes. Teach them the power of breath, the beauty of movement, and the gift of mindfulness.

I hope this book has inspired you to embrace the practice of Chair Yoga and all its transformative potential. If you would leave a review I will appreciate it very much.

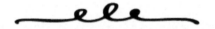

Chapter 12
About our Model

Sytske Kimman is the lovely lady you see in the photos. She has been regularly attending Yoga and Pilates lessons with me for the last 12 years. She is also an avid sailor and loves the ocean, the beach, and the outdoors in general.

Sytske also keeps active hiking. Unfortunately, she has recently been diagnosed with Leukemia. You may have noticed the band on her arm in all the photos which is covering a port for her chemotherapy. Sytske is doing as well as she can. She is both physically and mentally strong.

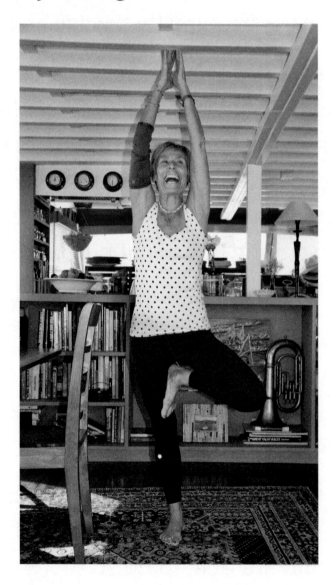

She has already undergone 5 chemotherapy rounds where she needs to go to the hospital for a week at a time.

Sytske does her Yoga and Pilates classes online from her Ward at the hospital when she is there. The doctors and nurses encourage this and they wait for her to finish her class sometimes before administering her drip if possible.

Send out your love to her as she undergoes her biggest challenge yet when she will be required to be in an isolation ward for 5 weeks (October/ November 2023).

This reminds us all how precious and sometimes fragile our health can be. Do what you are able to do so that you can invest in your health. I always imagine health like a bank account. When you do good things for your health, like exercising and eating well, you put money in your health bank account. When your activities include "bad" things like drinking too much coffee and alcohol, eating fatty foods, missing your workouts and allowing stress to govern your life, then you are taking money out of your health bank account.

Make sure your health bank account is looking abundant and then if you do experience any setbacks, like Sytske, you can deal with them all the better.

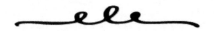

About the Author

Melinda Wright is a certified group exercise instructor, Personal Trainer, and Yoga and Pilates teacher. She specializes in working with people of all levels of fitness to provide safe and effective exercise sessions for them. She has developed ways of using Yoga, Pilates, and strength training to improve the well-being of her clients and help them to become healthier as they age. She makes it easy to learn any Yoga and Pilates exercise as she is encouraging and patient, using easy-to-understand explanations.

She helps people to feel good about themselves and their exercise sessions.

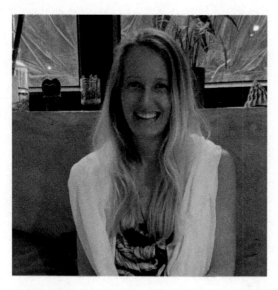

Melinda's life purpose is to help people of all ages learn and practice Yoga and Pilates regardless of any physical limitations they may have. She also instills in them a passion for these disciplines increasing their body-mind connection and leaving them feeling flexible, younger, and more energized.

Melinda has worked worldwide (South Africa, New Zealand, the United Kingdom, Hong Kong, and Australia) in health and fitness for more than 30 years.

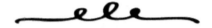

Also By

https://a.co/d/aiSS47O

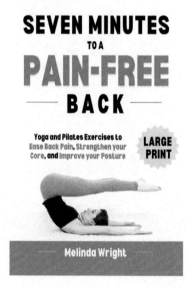

https://a.co/d/7qJucHp

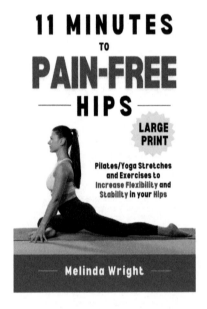

https://a.co/d/92rmQbU

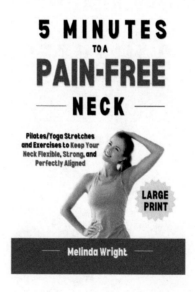

https://a.co/d/9sziopC

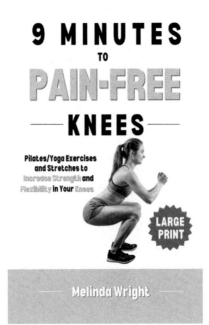

https://a.co/d/iQpCqJ6

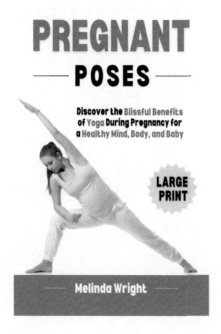

https://a.co/d/07TpMrV

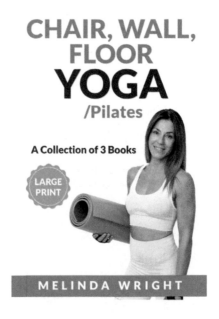

References

Brown, B. (2017). Braving the wilderness: the quest for true belonging and the courage to stand alone. Random House. U.S.

Chopra, D. (1994). The seven spiritual laws of success. New World Library/Amber–Allen Publishing. U.S

Dispenza, J. (2012). Breaking the habit of being yourself. Encephalon, Inc. U.S

Herdman, A. (2004). The Pilates directory. The Ivy Press Limited. U.K.

Iyengar, B.K.S. (1991). Light on yoga: the classic guide to yoga by the world's foremost authority. The Aquarian Press. U.K.

Lasater, J. (2005). Yoga abs. Rodmell Press.U.S.

Northrup, C. (2016). Making life easy. Hay House, Inc. U.S.

Pullig Schatz, M. (2016). Back care basics. Shambala. U.S.

Williams, A. (2020). Cleanse to heal: healing plans for sufferers of anxiety, depression, acne, eczema, Lyme, gut problems, weight issues, brain fog, migraines, bloating, vertigo, psoriasis, cysts, fatigue, PCOS, fibroids, UTI, endometriosis & autoimmune. Hay House Inc. U.S.

Acknowledgements

I am truly grateful to the following individuals who have provided me with help and support. Without them, this book would not be here.

Pauline Ching, my friend, editor, and accountability partner who checks in with me regularly.

Joan Bouttell, who selflessly takes time out of her busy life to take amazing photos and makes the sessions fun.

Our gorgeous model, Sytske Kimman, for making the poses look so good.

Tracey Godfrey for graciously providing her copyrighting skills.

Caroline Oliver, for your support and input. The world needs more compassionate doctors like you who are a good example of health and vitality.

Robyn Haddican, Emma Place, Sarah Fairhurst, Bart Kimman, and Diana Marchenko, who are regular clients in the studio, inspire me to keep daily classes running.

All my other clients, who have supported me throughout the years.

My friends, Kasia Stawiarska, Ralitsa Ivanova, Pebble Loh, and many more who support me.

The Medical Medium, for speaking the truth about healing and helping so many people who suffer from chronic illnesses.

My angels and guides, who lead me every day.

Mom and Dad, for all your love and support from afar.

My loving and supportive husband, Greg.

My beautiful daughter, Amy for being true to yourself and giving my life meaning.

I am truly grateful to you all. I appreciate all you add to my life!

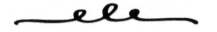